The Vibrant Cookin; Diet for Be;

Easy and Affordable Recipes to Los
Occasion

Demi Cooper

Table of contents

Grilled Cod Fillets with Lemon Dill Butter.. 6

Spicy Baked Shrimp 9

Shrimp and Cilantro Meal 11

The Original Dijon Fish.. 13

Lemony Garlic Shrimp 16

Brazilian Shrimp Stew 19

Inspiring Cajun Snow Crab 21

Grilled Lime Shrimp.. 24

Calamari Citrus 26

Spiced Up Salmon... 28

Chicken Piccata Stir-Fry 30

Ranch Meatballs 33

Beef Orzo with Feta 35

Light Beef Chili... 38

Mango Salsa 41

Watermelon Aguas Frescas 44

Chocolate Peanut Butter Banana Protein Shake.. 46

Skinny Pina Colada 48

Spindrift Grapefruit 50

Hearty Green Bean Roast... 51

Almond and Blistered Beans 53

Tomato Platter 56

Lemony Sprouts 58

Cool Garbanzo and Spinach Beans 61

Breakfast Super Antioxidant Berry Smoothie 63

Cucumber Tomato Surprise.. 65

Avocado Nori Rolls 67

Maple Ginger Pancakes.. 70

Chewy Chocolate Chip Cookies 74

Amazing Scrambled Turkey Eggs 76

Egg and Bacon Cups... 78

Pepperoni Omelet... 79

Cinnamon Baked Apple Chips 81

Herb and Avocado Omelet 84

Mustard Chicken 86

Chicken and Carrot Stew 88

The Delish Turkey Wrap 90

ALMOND BUTTERNUT CHICKEN 93

ZUCCHINI ZOODLES WITH CHICKEN AND BASIL.. 95

CRAZY LAMB SALAD 97

HEARTY ROASTED CAULIFLOWER 100

COOL CABBAGE FRIED BEEF... 103

FENNEL AND FIGS LAMB 105

BLACK BERRY CHICKEN WINGS.. 107

Grilled Cod Fillets with Lemon Dill Butter

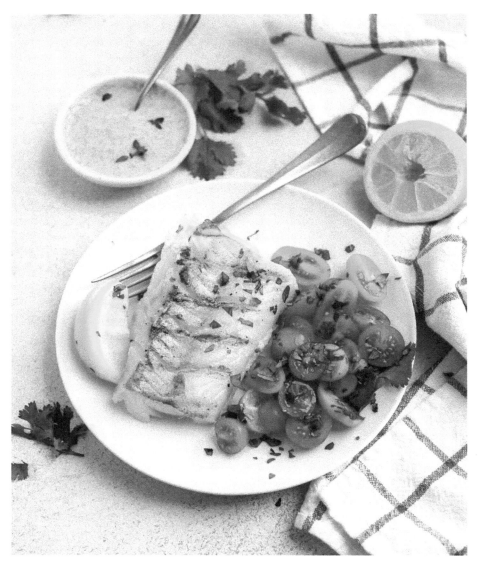

SmartPoints value: Green plan - 3SP, Blue plan - 2SP, Purple plan - 2SP

Total Time: 25 min, Prep time: 15 min, Cooking time: 10 min, Serves: 4

Nutritional value: Calories - 318.7g, Carbs - 6.7g, Fat - 13.0g, Protein - 41.7g

Grill the fish on slices of lemon topped with dill to add a delicious flavor to this dish. Become confident at grilling fish. With the layer of lemon slices, you can easily prevent the fish from sticking to the grate. To make use of a stovetop, prepare a grill pan by preheating it over medium-high heat until it is almost smoking, then continue with the recipe. The mixture of lemon, butter, and dill creates a robust sauce that becomes ready in minutes, even though it tastes like you spent hours preparing it. It is preferable to serve this dish with grilled asparagus.

Ingredients

- Olive oil -2 tsp
- Uncooked Atlantic cod - 24 oz, or another firm white fish like
- tilapia (four 6-oz fillets)
- Table salt - ½ tsp
- Lemon(s) (sliced 1/4-in thick) - 2 medium (you'll need 12 slices total)
- Dill - 2 tsp, chopped
- Dill - 4 sprig(s)
- Light butter - 4 tsp (at room temp.)

- Lemon zest - 1 tsp

Instructions

1.   Get your grill ready by preheating to medium-high heat. Continue the heating for at least 10 minutes after it reaches the desired temperature, then scrape the grate clean with a steel brush and coat it lightly with oil.

2.   While the grill heats up, pat the fish dry and sprinkle salt on it.

3.   Place three lemon slices on the grill carefully, overlapping slightly, and top it with a dill sprig and fish fillet.

4.   Repeat the same with the remaining lemon, dill, and fish. Cover the grill and cook without turning for 8-10 minutes until the fish is opaque all the way through and yields easily to a thin-bladed knife.

5.   While the cooking is on-going, mix the butter, chopped dill, and zest in a small shallow bowl.

6.   Transfer each lemon-dill-fish portion to a plate using two thin-bladed spatulas and top them with 1 1/2 tsp of lemon-dill butter and serve (serving the lemon slices is optional).

Spicy Baked Shrimp

Serving: 4

Prep Time: 10 minutes

Cook Time: 25 minutes + 2-4 hours

Ingredients:

- ½ ounce large shrimp, peeled and deveined
- Cooking spray as needed
- 1 teaspoon low sodium coconut amines
- 1 teaspoon parsley
- ½ teaspoon olive oil
- ½ tablespoon honey
- 1 tablespoon lemon juice

How To:

1.   Pre-heat your oven to 450 degrees F.

2.   Take a baking dish and grease it well.

3.   Mix altogether the ingredients and toss.

4.   Transfer to oven and bake for 8 minutes until shrimp turns pink.

5.   Serve and enjoy!

Nutrition (Per Serving)

Calories: 321

Fat: 9g

Carbohydrates: 44g

Protein: 22g

Shrimp and Cilantro Meal

Serving: 4

Prep Time: 10 minutes

Cook Time: 5 minutes

Ingredients:

- ¾ pounds shrimp, deveined and peeled
- tablespoons fresh lime juice
- ¼ teaspoon cloves, minced
- ½ teaspoon ground cumin
- 1 tablespoon olive oil
- 1 ¼ cups fresh cilantro, chopped
- 1 teaspoon lime zest
- ½ teaspoon sunflower seeds
- ¼ teaspoon pepper

Direction

1.   Take an outsized sized bowl and add shrimp, cumin, garlic, juice , ginger and toss well.

2.   Take an outsized sized non-stick skillet and add oil, allow the oil to

heat up over medium-high heat.

3.   Add shrimp mixture and sauté for 4 minutes.

4.   Remove the warmth and add cilantro, lime zest, sunflower seeds, and pepper.

5.   Mix well and serve hot!

Nutrition (Per Serving)

Calories: 177

Fat: 6g

Carbohydrates: 2g

Protein: 27g

The Original Dijon Fish

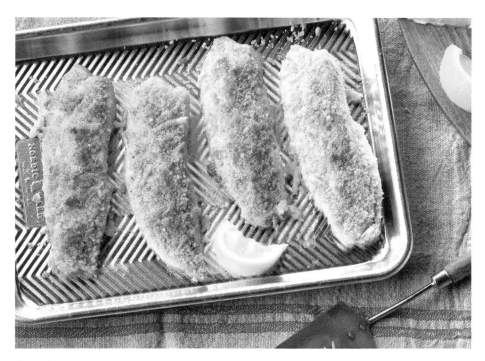

Serving: 2

Prep Time: 3 minutes

Cook Time: 12 minutes

Ingredients:

- 1 perch, flounder or sole fish florets
- 1 tablespoon Dijon mustard

- 1 ½ teaspoons lemon juice

- teaspoon low sodium Worcestershire sauce, low sodium

- tablespoons Italian seasoned bread crumbs

- 1 almond butter flavored cooking spray

How To:

1.   Preheat your oven to 450 degrees F.

2.   Take an 11 x 7-inch baking dish and arrange your fillets carefully.

3.   Take a little sized bowl and add juice, Worcester sauce, mustard and blend it well.

4.   Pour the combination over your fillet.

5.   Sprinkle an honest amount of breadcrumbs.

6.   Bake for 12 minutes until fish flakes off easily.

7.   Cut the fillet in half portions and enjoy!

Nutrition (Per Serving)

Calories: 125

Fat: 2g

Carbohydrates: 6g

Protein: 21g

Lemony Garlic Shrimp

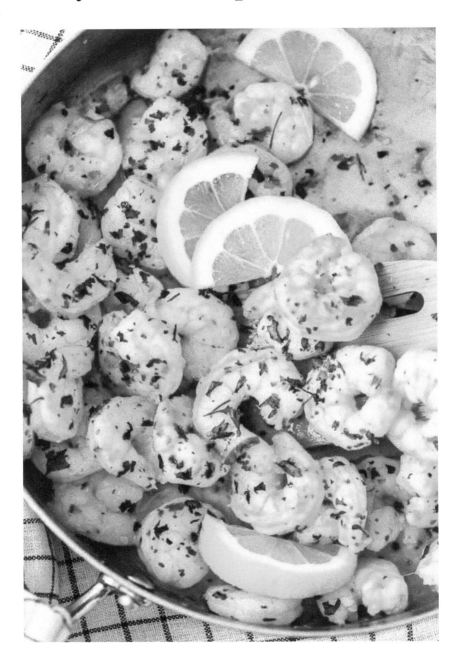

Serving: 4

Prep Time: 5-10 minutes

Cook Time: 10-15 minutes

Ingredients:

- 1 ¼ pounds shrimp, boiled or steamed
- tablespoons garlic, minced
- ¼ cup lemon juice
- tablespoons olive oil
- ¼ cup parsley

How To:

1.   Take alittle skillet and place over medium heat, add garlic and oil and stir-cook for 1 minute.

2.   Add parsley, juice and season with sunflower seeds and pepper accordingly.

3.   Add shrimp during a large bowl and transfer the mixture from the skillet over the shrimp.

4.   Chill and serve.

5.   Enjoy!

Nutrition (Per Serving)

Calories: 130

Fat: 3g

Carbohydrates:2g

Protein:22g

Brazilian Shrimp Stew

Serving: 4

Prep Time: 20 minutes

Cook Time: 25 minutes

Ingredients:

- Tablespoons lime juice
- 1 ½ tablespoons cumin, ground
- ½ tablespoons paprika
- ½ teaspoons garlic, minced
- ½ teaspoons pepper
- Pounds tilapia fillets, cut into bits
- 1 large onion, chopped
- Large bell peppers, cut into strips
- 1 can (14 ounces) tomato, drained
- 1 can (14 ounces) coconut milk
- handful of cilantros, chopped

How To:

1.   Take a large sized bowl and add lime juice, cumin, paprika, garlic, pepper and mix well.

2.   Add tilapia and coat it up.

3.   Cover and allow to marinate for 20 minutes.

4.   Set your Instant Pot to Sauté mode and add olive oil.

5.   Add onions and cook for 3 minutes until tender.

6.   Add pepper strips, tilapia, and tomatoes to a skillet.

7.   Pour coconut milk and cover, simmer for 20 minutes.

8.   Add cilantro during the final few minutes.

9.   Serve and enjoy!

Nutrition (Per Serving)

Calories: 471

Fat: 44g

Carbohydrates: 13g

Protein: 12g

Inspiring Cajun Snow Crab

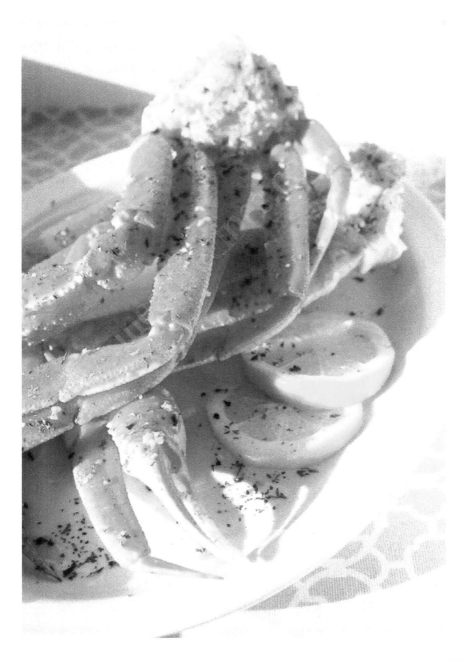

Serving: 2

Prep Time: 10 minutes

Cook Time: 10 minutes

Ingredients:

- 1 lemon, fresh and quartered tablespoons
- Cajun seasoning
- Bay leaves
- Snow crab legs, precooked and defrosted
- Golden ghee

How To:

1. Take a large pot and fill it about halfway with sunflower seeds and water.

2. Bring the water to a boil.

3. Squeeze lemon juice into the pot and toss in remaining lemon quarters.

4. Add bay leaves and Cajun seasoning.

5. Season for 1 minute.

6. Add crab legs and boil for 8 minutes (make sure to keep them submerged the whole time).

7. Melt ghee in microwave and use as dipping sauce, enjoy!

Nutrition (Per Serving)

Calories: 643

Fat: 51g

Carbohydrates: 3g

Protein: 41g

Grilled Lime Shrimp

Serving: 8

Prep Time: 25 minutes

Cook Time: 5 minutes

Ingredients:

- 1-pound medium shrimp, peeled and deveined
- 1 lime, juiced
- ½ cup olive oil
- Cajun seasoning

How To:

1.   Take a re-sealable zip bag and add lime juice, Cajun seasoning, olive oil.

2.   Add shrimp and shake it well, let it marinate for 20 minutes.

3.   Pre-heat your outdoor grill to medium heat.

4.   Lightly grease the grate.

5.   Remove shrimp from marinade and cook for 2 minutes per side.

6.   Serve and enjoy!

Nutrition (Per Serving)

Calories: 188

Fat: 3g

Net Carbohydrates: 1.2g

Protein: 13g

Calamari Citrus

Serving: 4

Prep Time: 10 minutes

Cook Time: 5 minutes

Ingredients:

- 1 lime, sliced
- lemon, sliced
- Pounds calamari tubes and tentacles, sliced
- Pepper to taste
- ¼ cup olive oil
- garlic cloves, minced
- tablespoons lemon juice
- orange, peeled and cut into segments
- tablespoons cilantro, chopped

How To:

1.   Take a bowl and add calamari, pepper, lime slices, lemon slices, orange slices, garlic, oil, cilantro, lemon juice and toss well.

2.   Take a pan and place it over medium-high heat.

3.   Add calamari mix and cook for 5 minutes.

4.   Divide into bowls and serve.

5.   Enjoy!

Nutrition (Per Serving)

Calories: 190

Fat: 2g

Net Carbohydrates: 11g

Protein: 14g

Spiced Up Salmon

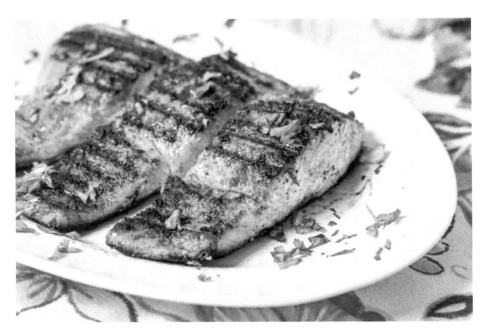

Serving: 4

Prep Time: 10 minutes

Cook Time: 10 minutes

Ingredients:

- Salmon fillets
- 2 tablespoons olive oil
- 1 teaspoon cumin, ground
- 1 teaspoon sweet paprika
- 1 teaspoon chili powder

- ½ teaspoon garlic powder
- Pinch of pepper

How To:

1.   Take a bowl and add cumin, paprika, onion, chili powder, garlic powder, pepper and toss well.

2.   Rub the salmon in the mixture.

3.   Take a pan and place it over medium heat, add oil and let it heat up.

4.   Add salmon and cook for 5 minutes, both sides.

5.   Divide between plates and serve.

6.   Enjoy!

Nutrition (Per Serving)

Calories: 220

Fat: 10g

Net Carbohydrates: 8g

Protein: 10g

Chicken Piccata Stir-Fry

SmartPoints value: Green plan - 4SP, Blue plan - 2SP, Purple plan - 2SP

Total Time: 25 min, Prep time: 20 min, Cooking time: 5 min, Serves: 4

Nutritional value: Cal - 190.5, Carbs - 5.6g, Fat - 9.4g, Protein - 18.6g

This dish is a combination of the classic Italian chicken piccata and Asian stir-fry.

Ingredients

- Black pepper (freshly ground) - ¼ tsp
- Capers (rinsed)- 1 Tbsp
- Chicken broth (fat-free) - ½ cup(s)
- Cornstarch (divided) - 2 tsp
- Dry sherry (divided)- 3 Tbsp
- Table salt (divided) - ¾ tsp
- Soy sauce (low sodium) - 1 Tbsp
- Peanut oil (divided) - 4 tsp, or vegetable oil
- Uncooked chicken breast (boneless, skinless) - 1 pound(s), cut into quarter-inch-thick slices

- Uncooked shallot(s) - 1 medium, thinly sliced Minced arlic - 1 Tbsp

- String beans (uncooked) - 2 cup(s), cut into two-inch lengths Parsley (fresh, chopped) - 2 Tbsp

- Lemon(s) - ½ medium, cut into four

Instructions

1.   Prepare a clean medium-sized bowl and mix chicken, 1 tsp of cornstarch,1 Tbsp of dry sherry,1/2 tsp salt, and pepper in it.

2.   Next, get a small bowl and combine broth, soy sauce, remaining 2 Tbsp of dry sherry, and 1 tsp of cornstarch.

3.   Preheat a fourteen-inch flat-bottomed wok or twelve-inch skillet over high heat to the point where a drop of water will evaporate within 1 to 2 seconds of contact, then swirl in one Tbsp oil.

4.   Add shallots and garlic, then stir-fry for 10 seconds. Push the shallot mixture to the sides of the wok and add the chicken, then spread in one layer in the wok.

5.   Cook the chicken undisturbed for 60 seconds, allowing the chicken to begin searing, then stir-fry another 60 seconds until chicken is no longer pink but not yet thoroughly cooked.

6.   Swirl the chicken in the remaining 1 tsp oil and toss in green beans and capers. Sprinkle on the remaining 1/4 tsp of salt and stir-fry for 30 seconds or until just combined.

7.   Swirl the chicken in the broth mixture and stir-fry for 1-2 minutes or until the chicken is cooked through, with the sauce slightly thickened.

8.   Sprinkle the parsley on it and serve with lemon wedges.

Ranch Meatballs

SmartPoints value: Green plan - 4SP, Blue plan - 4SP, Purple plan – 5SP

Total Time: 20mins, Prep time: 10 mins, Cooking time: 30mins, Serves: 4

Nutritional value: Calories - 195, Carbs - 6g, Fat - 6g, Protein - 26g

Meatball recipes are delicious protein recipes that are so satisfying and tasty. They can be a fun and easy meal. It becomes easier to prepare the perfect sized meatballs using a meatball shaper.

Ingredients

- Ground beef (96/4) (extra lean) - 1 lb
- Panko breadcrumbs - 1/3 cup(s)
- Egg substitute (Liquid, like egg beaters) - 1/4 cup
- Olive oil - 1 tsp
- Onion powder - 1 tbsp
- Garlic powder - 1 tbsp
- Dill (dried) - 2 tsp

- Parsley (dried) - 2 tsp

- Basil (dried) - 2 tsp

- Salt and pepper - Add to taste

Instructions

1.   Combine all the ingredients by hand in a large bowl and shape it into about 24 meatballs.

2.   Apply heat to the oil in a large non-stick skillet over medium-high heat.

3.   Place meatballs in the pan and cook for about 1-2 minutes on each side, until all sides get lightly browned.

4.   Reduce the heat to medium-low and pour in half a cup of water. Cover it and cook, occasionally stirring, until meatballs cook thoroughly; about 10-12 minutes.

Note: Meatballs are a perfect simple Weight Watchers dinner recipe for those who are watching Points but also savour the flavour

Beef Orzo with Feta

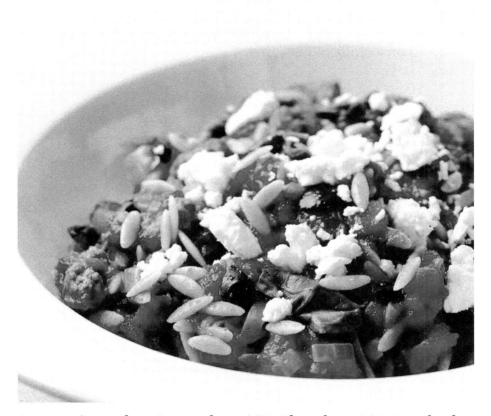

SmartPoints value: Green plan - 8SP, Blue plan - 8SP, Purple plan – 8SP

Total Time: 35mins, Prep time: 10mins, Cooking time: 25mins, Serves: 6

Nutritional value: Calories - 325, Carbs – 44g, Fat – 5.5g, Protein – 25g

Beef Orzo is one of those types of meals that you'll love to prepare now and then. The instructions for preparation are quite easy to follow, and the meal is just delicious. If you haven't tried it, you are missing out big time. You should give it a try for your next family dinner or friends gathering. This most satisfying weight-watching dinner recipe is perfect for warming you and your family up on a chilly fall evening.

Ingredients

- Ground beef (extra-lean) - 1 lb
- Whole wheat orzo - 10 oz
- Onion (finely chopped) - 1 large
- Garlic (minced) - 4 cloves
- Cinnamon (ground) - 1 tsp
- Oregano (dried) - 2 tsp
- Can tomatoes (crushed) - One 26oz
- Reduced-fat feta cheese (crumbled) - 1/3 cup
- Salt & pepper - Add to taste

Instructions

1.   Prepare whole orzo wheat according to package directions. Drain it and set aside.

2.   While the wheat is cooking, spray a large skillet with nonfat cooking spray, and set it over medium-high heat. Toss in some beef and cook until it mostly cooks through.

3.   Put in onions, oregano, garlic, cinnamon, salt, and pepper. Sauté the dish until the onions are tender and the beef cooks all the way through.

4.   Pour the crushed tomatoes into the skillet with the beef mixture, and cook on medium heat. Continue to cook, while occasionally stirring, until the mixture thickens; about 15 minutes.

5.   Dish the beef sauce with orzo and place in serving bowls. Top each bowl with 1 tbsp of feta.

Light Beef Chili

SmartPoints value: Green plan - 4SP, Blue plan - 4SP, Purple plan – 4SP

Total Time: 2hrs 30mins, Prep time: 30mins, Cooking time: 2hrs, Serves: 8

Nutritional value: Calories - 187, Carbs – 24g, Fat – 3g, Protein – 16g

This red meat dish is perfect for warming up on a chilly day. One of the reasons I love it is because preparing it is very easy. Often, I will make this chili, then measure and place each of them in a Ziploc bag and refrigerate. Whenever I need something hot and filling, all I need to do is grab one and microwave.

Ingredients

- Beef bouillon powder - 1 tbsp
- Bell pepper (red, diced) - 1 small
- Black pepper - 1/2 tsp
- Brewed coffee (strong) - 1 cup
- Chili powder - 3 tbsp
- Cocoa (unsweetened) - 1 tsp
- Cumin - 2 tbsp
- Dark beer - One 12oz can

- Garlic (minced) - 4 cloves
- Green pepper (diced) - 1 small
- Ground beef (extra lean) - 1 lb
- Kidney beans - One 15oz can
- Onion (diced) - 1 large
- Oregano - 2 tsp
- Paprika - 1 tsp
- Salt - 1 tsp
- Sugar - 1 tbsp
- Tomatoes (diced) - One 28oz can
- Tomato sauce - One 8oz can

Instructions

1. Place a large pot or Dutch oven over medium-high heat and spray it with non-fat cooking spray.

2. Add the onions and garlic, then cook until onions start to soften; about 3 minutes.

3. Toss in the ground beef and cook until the meat turns brown.

4. Add the diced bell peppers to the beef and cook for another 5 minutes.

5. Put in all the remaining ingredients asides the kidney beans and stir.

6.   Bring the content of the pot to a simmer, then stir in the kidney beans.

7.   Reduce the heat to medium-low, cover the pot, and let it cook for about 2 hours.

This perfect hearty beef chili made with extra lean ground beef simmers in fantastic spices and flavors to give you a desirable taste.

Mango Salsa

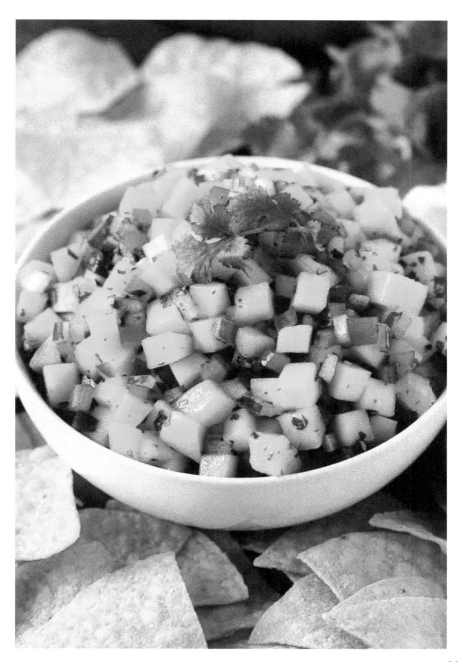

SmartPoints value: Green plan - 0SP, Blue plan - 0SP, Purple plan - 0SP

Total time: 15 min, Prep time: 15 min, Cooking time: 0 min, Serves: 4

Nutritional value: Calories – 71, Carbs – 17.7g, Fat – 0.5g, Protein – 1.3g

The mango salsa is a great snack full of fruits and veggies. Although salsa goes well with chips, it doesn't mean that you can use it for other things. However, it's an excellent topper for fish, chicken, and even salads.

Ingredients

Large mango (peeled and diced) - 1 item

- Red onion (finely chopped) - 1/2
- Red bell pepper (chopped) - 1 cup
- Jalapeno pepper (seeded and chopped) - (1 small piece)
- Garlic (minced) - 2 cloves
- Lime juice - 1 cup

- Pinch of salt (add to taste)

Instructions

1.   Put all the ingredients in a bowl and season as desired with salt.

2.   This mouthwatering sweet and savory salsa awakens your taste buds with delicious flavors. It is fresh, light, and loaded with antioxidants that make it a great pair with tortilla chips.

Watermelon Aguas Frescas

SmartPoints value: 3SP

Total time: 5 min, Prep time: 5 min, Serves - 4

Nutritional value: Calories - 57, Carbs - 14g, Fat - 0g, Protein - 1g

This pure Mexican blend of watermelon, lime juice, water, and a little sugar produces a delightful means of quenching thirst for Weight Watchers on a summer afternoon. You can find an alternative for the cantaloupe if you like.

Ingredients

- Watermelon (seedless, ripe; make sure it's nice and sweet) - 4 cups cubed
- Sugar (honey or agave nectar as an alternative) - 1 tbsp (or to taste)
- Water - 3 cups
- Lime juice (fresh) - 2-3 tsps.
- Mint (fresh) for garnish, if you desire

Instructions

1.   Put the cubed watermelon in a blender and add 1-1/2 cups of the water, the lime juice, and the sugar. Blend everything at high speed until smooth.

2.   Sieve the liquid blend through a medium strainer into a large pitcher (or bowl).

3.   Pour in the remaining 1-1/2 cups of water and stir.

4.   Chill in a refrigerator for 1 hour or longer, depending on the temperature you like.

5.   Drop a few cubes of ice in a glass and pour in the watermelon agua fresca.

6.   Add a mint sprig to garnish if you desire.

Chocolate Peanut Butter Banana Protein Shake

SmartPoints value: 6SP

Total time: 5 min, Prep time: 5 min, Serves: 1

Nutritional value: Calories - 299, Carbs - 29.6g, Fat - 6.1g, Protein - 36.2g

This drink provides a fast, healthy, and delicious way to begin your day, packed with protein to help keep you satisfied until lunchtime.

Ingredients

- Cottage cheese (non-fat) - 1/2 cup
- Peanut Butter Flour (PB2) - 2 tablespoons
- Chocolate protein powder - 1 scoop
- Banana (frozen) - 1/2 finger
- A handful of ice cubes
- Sweetener - to taste (You may not need this if your protein powder already has sweetener in it)

Instructions

1.   Mix all the ingredients in a blender and process until you get a smooth mixture.

2.   You can add more ice cubes to give a thicker consistency to the protein shake.

3.   You can use less ice if you want your drink to be thinner. Add more water.

Skinny Pina Colada

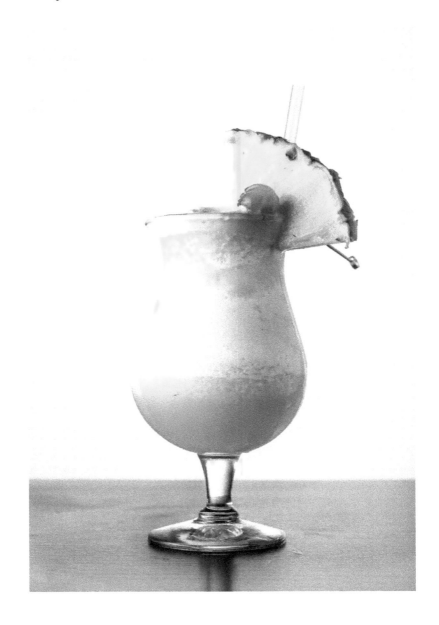

SmartPoints - 7SP

Total time: 5 min, Prep time: 5 min, Serves: 1

Nutritional value: Calories - 183, Carbs - 11g, Fat - 0.5g, Protein - 9.5g

This drink recipe is a cleaned-up version of a pina colada from the Weight Watchers, thickened with vanilla protein powder instead of the cream of coconut. This satisfying and sweet drink has just 7 SmartPoints, which is about 1/3 of the points of a traditional Pina Colada.

Ingredients

- Vanilla protein powder with about 100 calories per 1-ounce serving (natural) - 3 tablespoons
- Crushed pineapple packed in juice (canned, not drained) - 1/4 cup
- White rum - 1 -1/2 ounces
- Coconut extract - 1/8 teaspoon
- Crushed ice, about eight ice cubes - 1 cup

Instructions

1.   Put all the ingredients in a blender.

2.   Pour in half a cup of water, and blend at high speed until it is smooth.

Spindrift Grapefruit

SmartPoints value: 1SP

Serving size - 355ml

Nutritional value: Calories - 17, Carbs - 4g, Fat - 0g, Protein - 0g

Spindrift is America's first sparkling water fruit drink.

The several varieties of the drink are all created from sparkling water and real squeezed fruits.

Aside from the grapefruit variety, the other types you can enjoy with your meal include blackberry, cucumber, lemon, raspberry lime, orange mango, strawberry, half & half, and cranberry raspberry.

Ingredients

The ingredients of Grapefruit drink include grapefruit juice, lemon juice, orange juice,

Hearty Green Bean Roast

Serving: 4

Prep Time: 10 minutes

Cook Time: 20 minutes

Ingredients:

- 1 whole egg
- 2 tablespoons olive oil
- Sunflower seeds and pepper to taste
- 1-pound fresh green beans
- 5 ½ tablespoons grated parmesan cheese

How To:

1. Pre-heat your oven to 400 degrees F.
2. Take a bowl and whisk in eggs with oil and spices.
3. Add beans and mix well.
4. Stir in parmesan cheese and pour the mix into baking pan (lined with parchment paper).
5. Bake for 15-20 minutes.
6. Serve warm and enjoy!

Nutrition (Per Serving)

Calories: 216

Fat: 21g

Carbohydrates: 7g

Protein: 9g

Almond and Blistered Beans

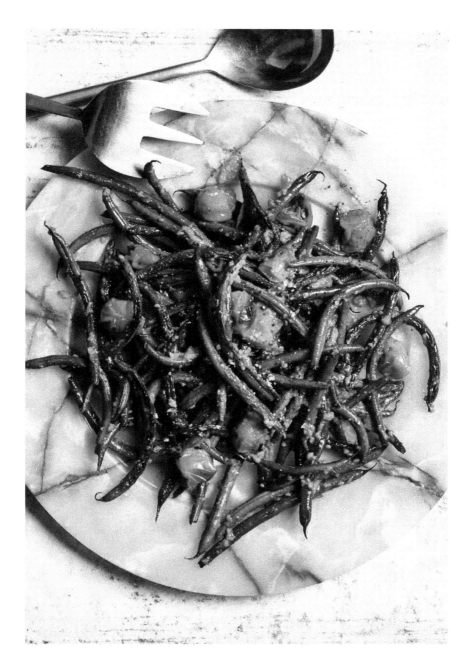

Serving: 4

Prep Time: 10 minutes

Cook Time: 20 minutes

Ingredients:

- 1-pound fresh green beans, ends trimmed
- 1 ½ tablespoon olive oil
- ¼ teaspoon sunflower seeds
- 1 ½ tablespoons fresh dill, minced
- Juice of 1 lemon
- ¼ cup crushed almonds
- Sunflower seeds as needed

How To:

1.   Pre-heat your oven to 400 degrees F.

2.   Add the green beans with your olive oil and also the sunflower seeds.

3.   Then spread them in one single layer on a large sized sheet pan.

4.   Roast it for 10 minutes and stir, then roast for another 8-10 minutes.

5.   Remove from the oven and keep stirring in the lemon juice alongside the dill.

6.   Top it with crushed almonds and some flaked sunflower seeds and serve.

Nutrition (Per Serving)

Calories: 347

Fat: 16g

Carbohydrates: 6g

Protein: 45g

Tomato Platter

Serving: 8

Prep Time: 10 minutes + Chill time

Cook Time: Nil

Ingredients:

- 1/3 cup olive oil
- 1 teaspoon sunflower seeds
- 2 tablespoons onion, chopped
- ¼ teaspoon pepper
- ½ a garlic, minced
- 1 tablespoon fresh parsley, minced
- 3 large fresh tomatoes, sliced
- 1 teaspoon dried basil
- ¼ cup red wine vinegar

How To:

1.   Take a shallow dish and arrange tomatoes in the dish.

2.   Add the rest of the ingredients in a mason jar, cover the jar and shake it well.

3.   Pour the mix over tomato slices.

4.   Let it chill for 2-3 hours.

5.   Serve!

Nutrition (Per Serving)

Calories: 350

Fat: 28g

Carbohydrates: 10g

Protein: 14g

Lemony Sprouts

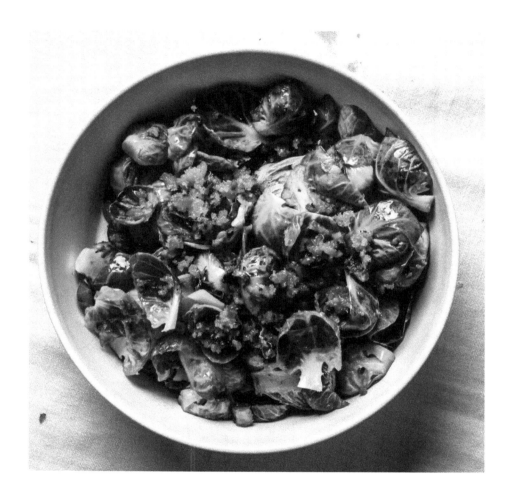

Serving: 4

Prep Time: 10 minutes

Cook Time: Nil

Ingredients:

- 1 pound Brussels sprouts, trimmed and shredded
- 8 tablespoons olive oil
- 1 lemon, juice and zested
- Sunflower seeds and pepper to taste
- ¾ cup spicy almond and seed mix

How To:

1.   Take a bowl and mix in lemon juice, sunflower seeds, pepper and olive oil.

2.   Mix well.

3.   Stir in shredded Brussels sprouts and toss.

4.   Let it sit for 10 minutes.

5.   Add nuts and toss.

6.   Serve and enjoy!

Nutrition (Per Serving)

Calories: 382

Fat: 36g

Carbohydrates: 9g

Protein: 7g

Cool Garbanzo and Spinach Beans

Serving: 4

Prep Time: 5-10 minutes

Cook Time: Nil

Ingredients:

- 1 tablespoon olive oil
- ½ onion, diced
- 10 ounces spinach, chopped
- 12 ounces garbanzo beans
- ½ teaspoon cumin

How To:

1.   Take a skillet and add olive oil, let it warm over medium-low heat.

2.   Add onions, garbanzo and cook for 5 minutes.

3.   Stir in spinach, cumin, garbanzo beans and season with sunflower seeds.

4.   Use a spoon to smash gently.

5.   Cook thoroughly until heated, enjoy!

Nutrition (Per Serving)

Calories: 90

Fat: 4g

Carbohydrates:11g

Protein:4g

Breakfast Super Antioxidant Berry Smoothie

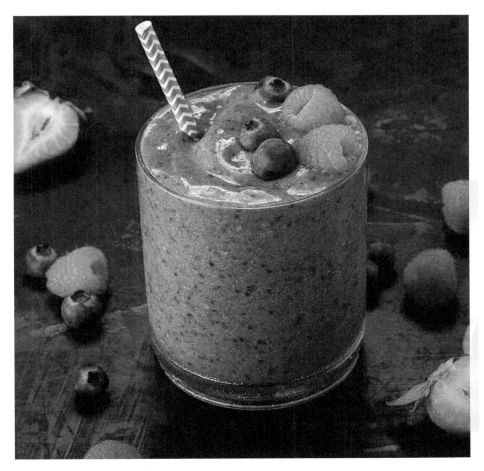

servings per container - 5

Prep Total - 10 min

Serving Size - 4 cup (20g)

Nutritional Facts

Total Fat 2g

Sodium 7mg

Total Carbohydrate 20g

Protein 3g

Ingredients

- 1 cup of filtered water
- 1 whole orange, peeled, de-seeded & cut into chunks
- 2 cups frozen raspberries or blackberries
- 1 Tablespoon goji berries
- 1 1/2 Tablespoons hemp seeds or plant-based protein powder
- 2 cups leafy greens (parsley, spinach, or kale)

Instructions:

1. Blend on high until smooth
2. Serve and drink immediately

Cucumber Tomato Surprise

servings per container - 5

Prep Total - 10 min

Serving Size 2/3 cup (55g)

Nutritional Facts

Total Fat 20g

Total Carbohydrate 14g

Total Sugar 2g

Protein 7g

Ingredients

- Chopped 1 medium of tomato
- 1 small cucumber peeled in stripes and chopped
- 1 large avocado cut into cubes
- 1 half of a lemon or lime squeezed
- ½1 tsp. Himalayan or Real salt
- 1 Teaspoon of original olive oil, MCT or coconut oil

Instructions:

1. Mix everything together and enjoy

2. This dish tastes even better after sitting for 40 – 60 minutes

3. Blend into a soup if desired.

Avocado Nori Rolls

Nutritional Facts

servings per container 10

Prep Total 10 min

Serving Size 2/3 cup (70g)

Amount per serving 15

Calories

% Daily Value

Total Fat 2g 10%

Saturated Fat 1g 9%

Trans Fat 10g -

Cholesterol 1%

Sodium 70mg 5%

Total Carbohydrate 22g 40%

Dietary Fiber 4g 2%

Total Sugar 12g -

Protein 3g

Vitamin C 2mcg 2%

Calcium 260mg 7%

Iron 8mg 2%

Potassium 235mg 4%

Ingredients

- 2 sheets of raw or toasted sushi nori
- 1 large Romaine leaf cut in half down the length of the spine
- 2 Teaspoon of spicy miso paste
- 1 avocado, peeled and sliced
- ½ red, yellow or orange bell pepper, julienned
- ½ cucumber, peeled, seeded and julienned
- ½ cup raw sauerkraut
- ½ carrot, beet or zucchini, shredded
- 1 cup alfalfa or favorite green sprouts
- 1 small bowl of water for sealing roll

Instructions:

1.   Place a sheet of nori on a sushi rolling mat or washcloth, lining it up at the end closest to you.

2.   Place the Romaine leaf on the edge of the nori with the spine closest to you.

3.   Spread Spicy Miso Paste on the Romaine

4.   Line the leaf with all ingredients in descending order, placing

sprouts on last

5.   Roll the Nori sheet away from you, tucking the ingredients in with your fingers, and seal the roll with water or Spicy Miso Paste. Slice the roll into 6 or 8 rounds.

Maple Ginger Pancakes

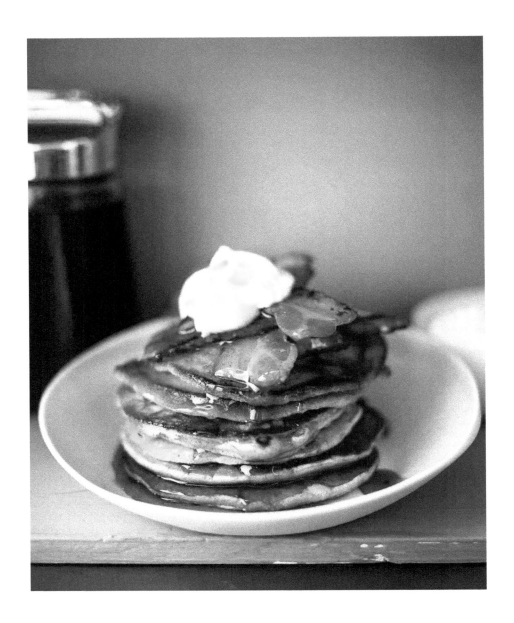

Nutritional Facts

servings per container 4

Prep Total 10 min

Serving Size 2/3 cup (20g)

Amount per serving 20

Calories

% Daily Value

Total Facts 10g 10%

Saturated Fat 0g 7%

Trans Fat 2g -

Cholesterol 3%

Sodium 10mg 2%

Total Carbohydrate 7g 3%

Dietary Fiber 2g 4%

Total Sugar 1g -

Protein 3g

Vitamin C 2mcg 10%

Calcium 260mg 20%

Iron 8mg 30%

Potassium 235mg 6%

Ingredients

- 1 or 2 cup flour
- 1 tablespoonful baking powder
- 1/2 tablespoonful kosher salt
- 1/4 tablespoonful ground ginger
- 1/4 table spoonful pumpkin pie spice
- 1/3 cup maple syrup
- 2/4 cup water

- minced 1/4 cup + 1 tablespoonful crystallized ginger slices together

Instructions:

1.   In a neat bowl mix together the first five recipes

2.   Add flour with syrup with water and stir together, after that add in the chopped ginger & stir until-just-combined.

3.   Heat your frying pan and coat with a nonstick cooking spray

4.   Pour in 1/4 cup of the batter and allow to heat until it form bubbles. Allow to cook until browned

5.   Serve warm & topped with a slathering of vegan butter, a splash of maple syrup, and garnished with chopped candied ginger.

Chewy Chocolate Chip Cookies

Nutritional Facts

servings per container   10

Prep Total   10 min

Serving Size 2/3 cup (40g)

Amount per serving 10

Calories

% Daily Value

Total Fat 10g 2%

Saturated Fat 1g   5%

Trans Fat 0g -

Cholesterol   15%

Sodium 120mg   8%

Total Carbohydrate 21g   10%

Dietary Fiber 4g   1%

Total Sugar 1g   0%

Protein 6g

Vitamin C 2mcg   7%

Calcium 210mg   51%

Iron 8mg   1%

Potassium 235mg   10%

Ingredients

- 1 cup vegan butter, softened
  - ½ cup white sugar
- ½ cup brown sugar
- ¼ cup dairy-free milk
- 1 teaspoon vanilla
- 2 ¼ cups flour
- ½ teaspoon salt
- 1 teaspoon baking soda
- 12 ounces dairy-free chocolate chips

Instructions:

1.   Preheat oven to 350°F.

2.   In a large bowl, mix the butter, white sugar, and brown sugar until light and fluffy. Slowly stir in the dairy-free milk and then add the vanilla to make a creamy mixture.

3.   In a separate bowl, combine the flour, salt, and baking soda.

4.   You need to add this dry mixture to the liquid mixture and stir well. Fold in the chocolate chips.

5.   Drop small spoonful of the batter onto non-stick cookie sheets and bake for 9 minutes.

Amazing Scrambled Turkey Eggs

Serving: 2

Prep Time: 15 minutes

Cook Time: 15 minutes

Ingredients:

- 1 tablespoon coconut oil
- 1 medium red bell pepper, diced
- ½ medium yellow onion, diced
- ¼ teaspoon hot pepper sauce
- 3 large free-range eggs
- ¼ teaspoon black pepper, freshly ground
- ¼ teaspoon salt

How To:

1. Set a pan to medium-high heat, add copra oil , let it heat up
2. Add onions and sauté.
3. Add turkey and red pepper .
4. Cook until the turkey is cooked.
5. Take a bowl and beat eggs, stir in salt and pepper.

6.   Pour eggs within the pan with turkey and gently cook and scramble eggs.

7.   Top with sauce and enjoy!

Nutrition (Per Serving)

Calories: 435

Fat: 30g

Carbohydrates: 34g

Protein: 16g

Egg and Bacon Cups

Serving: 6

Prep Time: 10 minutes

Cook Time: 15 minutes

Ingredients:

- 2 bacon strips
- 2 large eggs
- A handful of fresh spinach
- ¼ cup cheese
- Salt and pepper to taste

How To:

1.   Preheat your oven to 400 degrees F.

2.   Fry bacon during a skillet over medium heat, drain the oil and keep them on the side.

3.   Take muffin tin and grease with oil.

4.   Line with a slice of bacon, depress the bacon well, ensuring that the ends are protruding (to be used as handles).

5.   Take a bowl and beat eggs.

6.   Drain and pat the spinach dry.

7.   Add the spinach to the eggs.

8.   Add 1 / 4 of the mixture in each of your muffin tins.

9.   Sprinkle cheese and season.

10.   Bake for quarter-hour .

11.   Enjoy!

Nutrition (Per Serving)

Calories: 101

Fat: 7g

Carbohydrates: 2g

Protein: 8g

Fiber: 1g

Net Carbs: 1g

Pepperoni Omelet

Serving: 2

Prep Time: 5 minutes

Cook Time: 20 minutes

Ingredients:

- 3 eggs
- 7 pepperoni slices

- 1 teaspoon coconut cream
- Salt and freshly ground black pepper, to taste
- 1 tablespoons butter

How To:

1.   Take a bowl and whisk eggs with all the remaining ingredients in it.

2.   Then take a skillet and warmth the butter.

3.   Pour ¼ of the egg mixture into your skillet.

4.   After that, cook for two minutes per side.

5.   Repeat to use the whole batter.

6.   Serve warm and enjoy!

Nutrition (Per Serving)

Calories: 141

Fat: 11.5g

Carbohydrates: 0.6g

Protein: 8.9g

Cinnamon Baked Apple Chips

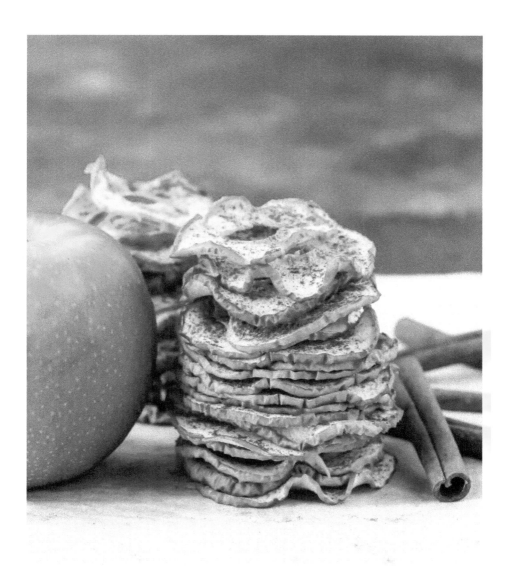

Serving: 2

Prep Time: 5 minutes

Cook Time: 2 hours

Ingredients:

- 1 teaspoon cinnamon
- 1-2 apples

How To:

1.   Preheat your oven to 200 degrees F.

2.   Take a pointy knife and slice apples into thin slices.

3.   Discard seeds.

4.   Line a baking sheet with parchment paper and arrange apples thereon .

5.   Confirm they are doing not overlap.

6.   Once done, sprinkle cinnamon over apples.

7.   Bake within the oven for 1 hour.

8.   Flip and bake for an hour more until not moist.

9.   Serve and enjoy!

Nutrition (Per Serving)

Calories: 147

Fat: 0g

Carbohydrates: 39g

Protein: 1g

Herb and Avocado Omelet

Serving: 2

 Prep Time: 2 minutes

Cook Time: 10 minutes

Ingredients:

- large free-range eggs
- ½ medium avocado, sliced
- ½ cup almonds, sliced
- Salt and pepper as needed

How To:

1.   Take a non-stick skillet and place it over medium-high heat.
2.   Take a bowl and add eggs, beat the eggs.
3.   Pour into the skillet and cook for 1 minute.
4.   Reduce heat to low and cook for 4 minutes.
5.   Top the omelet with almonds and avocado.
6.   Sprinkle salt and pepper and serve.
7.   Enjoy!

Nutrition (Per Serving)

Calories: 193

Fat: 15g

Carbohydrates: 5g

Protein: 10g

Mustard Chicken

Serving: 2

Prep Time: 10 minutes

Cook Time: 40 minutes

Ingredients:

- 2 chicken breasts
- 1/4 cup chicken broth
- 2 tablespoons mustard
- 1 1/2 tablespoons olive oil
- 1/2 teaspoon paprika
- 1/2 teaspoon chili powder
- 1/2 teaspoon garlic powder

How To:

1.   Take alittle bowl and blend mustard, olive oil, paprika, chicken stock , garlic powder, chicken stock , and chili.

2.   Add pigeon breast and marinate for half-hour .

3.   Take a lined baking sheet and arrange the chicken.

4.   Bake for 35 minutes at 375 degrees F.

5.   Serve and enjoy!

Nutrition (Per Serving)

Calories: 531

Fat: 23g

Carbohydrates: 10g

Protein: 64g

Chicken and Carrot Stew

Serving: 4

Prep Time: 15 minutes

Cook Time: 6 hours

Ingredients:

- 4 boneless chicken breast, cubed
- 3 cups of carrots, peeled and cubed
- 1 cup onion, chopped
- 1 cup tomatoes, chopped
- 1 teaspoon of dried thyme
- 2 cups of chicken broth
- 2 garlic cloves, minced
- Sunflower seeds and pepper as needed

How To:

1. Add all of the listed ingredients to a Slow Cooker.
2. Stir and shut the lid.
3. Cook for six hours.
4. Serve hot and enjoy!

Nutrition (Per Serving)

Calories: 182

Fat: 3g

Carbohydrates: 10g

Protein: 39g

The Delish Turkey Wrap

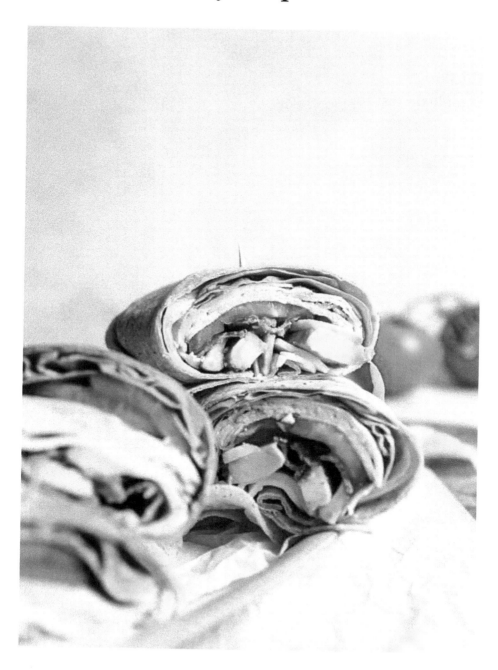

Serving: 6

Prep Time: 10 minutes

Cook Time: 10 minutes

Ingredients:

- 1 ¼ pounds ground turkey, lean
- 4 green onions, minced
- 1 tablespoon olive oil
- 1 garlic clove, minced
- 2 teaspoons chili paste
- 8-ounce water chestnut, diced
- 3 tablespoons hoisin sauce
- 2 tablespoon coconut aminos
- 1 tablespoon rice vinegar
- 12 almond butter lettuce leaves
- 1/8 teaspoon sunflower seeds

How To:

1. Take a pan and place it over medium heat, add turkey and garlic to the pan.

2. Heat for six minutes until cooked.

3. Take a bowl and transfer turkey to the bowl.

4. Add onions and water chestnuts.

5.   Stir in duck sauce , coconut aminos, vinegar and chili paste.

6.   Toss well and transfer mix to lettuce leaves.

7.   Serve and enjoy!

Nutrition (Per Serving)

Calories: 162

Fat: 4g

Net Carbohydrates: 7g

Protein: 23g

Almond butternut Chicken

Serving: 4

Prep Time: 15 minutes

Cook Time: 30 minutes

Ingredients:

- ½ pound Nitrate free bacon
- 6 chicken thighs, boneless and skinless
- 2-3 cups almond butternut squash, cubed
- Extra virgin olive oil Fresh chopped sage
- Sunflower seeds and pepper as needed

How To:

1.   Prepare your oven by preheating it to 425 degrees F.

2.   Take an outsized skillet and place it over medium-high heat, add bacon and fry until crispy.

3.   Take a slice of bacon and place it on the side, crumble the bacon.

4.   Add cubed almond butternut squash within the bacon grease and sauté, season with sunflower seeds and pepper.

5.   Once the squash is tender, remove skillet and transfer to a plate.

6. Add copra oil to the skillet and add chicken thighs, cook for 10 minutes.

7. Season with sunflower seeds and pepper.

8. Remove skillet from stove and transfer to oven.

9. Bake for 12-15 minutes, top with the crumbled bacon and sage.

10. Enjoy!

Nutrition (Per Serving)

Calories: 323

Fat: 19g

Carbohydrates: 8g

Protein: 12g

Zucchini Zoodles with Chicken and Basil

Serving: 3

Prep Time: 10 minutes

Cook Time: 10 minutes

Ingredients:

- 2 chicken fillets, cubed
- 2 tablespoons ghee
- 1-pound tomatoes, diced
- ½ cup basil, chopped
- ¼ cup almond milk
- 1 garlic clove, peeled, minced
- 1 zucchini, shredded

How To:

1.   Sauté cubed chicken in ghee until not pink.

2.   Add tomatoes and season with sunflower seeds.

3.   Simmer and reduce liquid.

4.   Prepare your zucchini Zoodles by shredding zucchini during a kitchen appliance .

5.   Add basil, garlic, coconut almond milk to the chicken and cook for a couple of minutes.

6.   Add half the zucchini Zoodles to a bowl and top with creamy tomato basil chicken.

7.   Enjoy!

Nutrition (Per Serving)

Calories: 540

Fat: 27g

Carbohydrates: 13g

Protein: 59g

Crazy Lamb Salad

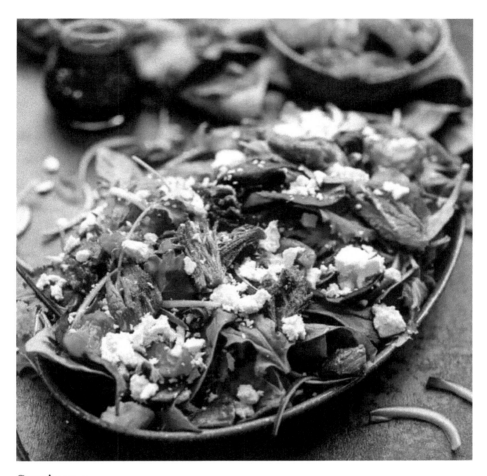

Serving: 4

Prep Time: 10 minutes

Cook Time: 35 minutes

Ingredients:

- 1 tablespoon olive oil
- 3 pound leg of lamb, bone removed, leg butterflied
- Salt and pepper to taste
- 1 teaspoon cumin
- Pinch of dried thyme
- 2 garlic cloves, peeled and minced For Salad
- 4 ounces feta cheese, crumbled
- ½ cup pecans
- 2 cups spinach
- 1 ½ tablespoons lemon juice
- ¼ cup olive oil
- 1 cup fresh mint, chopped

How To:

1.   Rub lamb with salt and pepper, 1 tablespoon oil, thyme, cumin, minced garlic.

2.   Pre-heat your grill to medium-high and transfer lamb.

3.   Cook for 40 minutes, ensuring to flip it once.

4.   Take a lined baking sheet and spread the pecans.

5.   Toast in oven for 10 minutes at 350 degree F.

6.   Transfer grilled lamb to chopping board and let it cool.

7.   Slice.

8.   Take a salad bowl and add spinach, 1 cup mint, feta cheese, ¼ cup vegetable oil , juice , toasted pecans, salt, pepper and toss well.

9.   Add lamb slices on top.

10.   Serve and enjoy!

Nutrition (Per Serving)

Calories: 334

Fat: 33g

Carbohydrates: 5g

Protein: 7g

Hearty Roasted Cauliflower

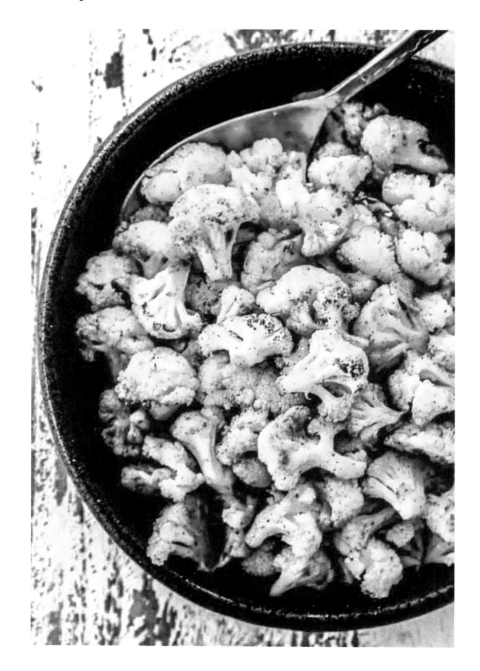

Serving: 8

Prep Time: 5 minutes

Cook Time: 30 minutes

Ingredients:

- 1 large cauliflower head
- 2 tablespoons melted coconut oil
- 2 tablespoons fresh thyme
- 1 teaspoon Celtic sea sunflower seeds
- 1 teaspoon fresh ground pepper
- 1 head roasted garlic
- 2 tablespoons fresh thyme for garnish

How To:

1. Pre-heat your oven to 425 degrees F.

2. Rinse cauliflower and trim, core and sliced.

3. Lay cauliflower evenly on rimmed baking tray.

4. Drizzle copra oil evenly over cauliflower, sprinkle thyme leaves .

5. Season with pinch of sunflower seeds and pepper.

6. Squeeze roasted garlic.

7.   Roast cauliflower until slightly caramelized for about half-hour , ensuring to show once.

8.   Garnish with fresh thyme leaves.

9.   Enjoy!

Nutrition (Per Serving)

Calories: 129

Fat: 11g

Carbohydrates: 6g

Protein: 7g

Cool Cabbage Fried Beef

Serving: 4

Prep Time: 5 minutes

Cook Time: 15 minutes

Ingredients:

- 1-pound beef, ground and lean
- ½ pound bacon
- 1 onion
- 1 garlic clove, minced
- ½ head cabbage
- pepper to taste

How To:

1. Take skillet and place it over medium heat.
2. Add chopped bacon, beef and onion until slightly browned.
3. Transfer to a bowl and keep it covered.
4. Add minced garlic and cabbage to the skillet and cook until slightly browned.
5. Return the bottom beef mix to the skillet and simmer for 3-5 minutes over low heat.
6. Serve and enjoy!

Nutrition (Per Serving)

Calories: 360

Fat: 22g

Net Carbohydrates: 5g

Protein: 34g

Fennel and Figs Lamb

Serving: 2

Prep Time: 10 minutes

Cook Time: 40 minutes

Ingredients:

- 6 ounces lamb racks 1 fennel bulbs, sliced pepper to taste
- 1 tablespoon olive oil
- 2 figs, cut in half
- 1/8 cup apple cider vinegar
- 1/2 tablespoon swerve

How To:

1.   Take a bowl and add fennel, figs, vinegar, swerve, oil and toss.

2.   Transfer to baking dish.

3.   Season with sunflower seeds and pepper.

4.   Bake for quarter-hour at 400 degrees F.

5.   Season lamb with sunflower seeds and pepper and transfer to a heated pan over medium-high heat.

6.   Cook for a couple of minutes.

7.   Add lamb to the baking dish with fennel and bake for 20 minutes.

8.   Divide between plates and serve.

9.   Enjoy!

Nutrition (Per Serving)

Calories: 230

Fat: 3g

Carbohydrates: 5g

Protein: 10g

Black Berry Chicken Wings

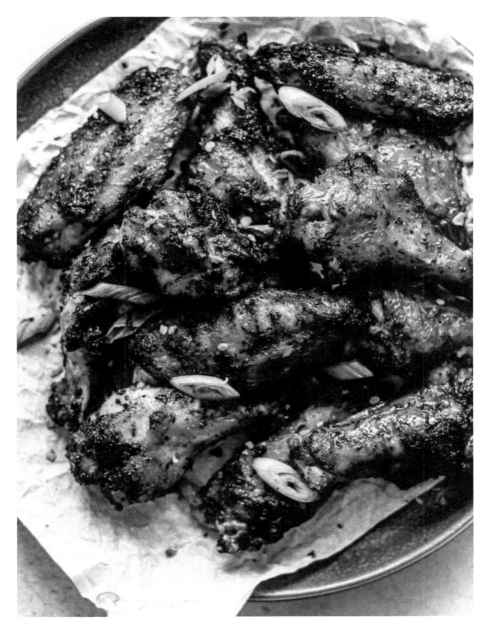

Serving: 4

Prep Time: 35 minutes

Cook Time: 50minutes

Ingredients:

- 3 pounds chicken wings, about 20 pieces
- ½ cup blackberry chipotle jam
- Pepper to taste
- ½ cup water

How To:

1. Add water and jam to a bowl and blend well.

2. Place chicken wings during a zip bag and add two-thirds of marinade.

3. Season with pepper.

4. Let it marinate for half-hour .

5. Pre-heat your oven to 400 degrees F.

6. Prepare a baking sheet and wire rack, place chicken wings in wire rack and bake for quarter-hour .

7. Brush remaining marinade and bake for half-hour more.

8. Enjoy!

Nutrition (Per Serving)

Calories: 502

Fat: 39g

Carbohydrates: 01.8g

Protein: 34g

Lightning Source UK Ltd.
Milton Keynes UK
UKHW020704130521
383649UK00005B/117